Pain Relief with Osteomassage

The Authors

Ronald M. Lawrence, M.D.

Dr. Lawrence is a founding member of the International Association for the Study of Pain, a member of the National Advisory Council on Aging, and a Medical Advisor to The President's Council on Physical Fitness and Sport. An Assistant Clinical Professor, Neuropsychiatric Institute, School of Medicine, University of California at Los Angeles, he is a diplomate of the American National Board of Psychiatry, the American Board of Family Practice, and the American Board of Electroencephalography, and Board Eligible in Neurology. He has for 28 years been engaged in medical practice in North Hollywood, California.

He holds or has held positions as President and Founder, American Medical Joggers Association; Director, National Jogging Association; Consultant, U.S. Olympic Committee; President, Acupuncture Medical Association of America; President, American Academy of Acupuncture Medicine; Secretary, American Academy of Sports Physicians; Director, American Technion Society; and others.

Among his awards are the Philip Noel Baker Research Award, United Nations (UNESCO), presented at the Montreal Olympics; Maimonides Award, American Technion Society; Peace Medal, Technion Medical School, Haifa, Israel; Research Associate, Rockefeller Institute for Medical Research, New York.

He has served as guest lecturer at Harvard University, Yale University, University of California, Tulane University and others. He holds numerous fellowships and memberships and is the author of 25 scientific papers in the fields of Pain, Neurophysiology, Cerebral Blood Flow, Electroencephalography, Sports Psychology, and Neurology.

Stanley Rosenberg

Stanley Rosenberg is founder, administrative leader, and teacher of Osteomassage at the Institute for Massage Therapy in Silkeborg, Denmark. He established the Hwa Yu Tai Chi Institute in Copenhagen. He has a broad background in spirit-body-mind disciplines. In theater he directed and taught at Yale School of Drama, the National Theater School of Denmark, and the National Academy of Dramatic Art in Iceland. He has served as a consultant to the United States National Rowing Team as World Champions. He has served as coach and teacher to United States and European television and motion picture celebrities.

Pain Relief with Osteomassage

At Your Fingertips: a Simple, New Method for Achieving Relaxation and Relief from Pain

By
Ronald M. Lawrence, M.D.
Assistant Clinical Professor, Neuropsychiatric Institute,
School of Medicine, University of California
at Los Angeles

Stanley Rosenberg
Founder, Tai Chi Institute of Copenhagen

Woodbridge Press/Santa Barbara, California

Photography: Ejler Neergaard
Model: Britta Hyldequist

Published and distributed by

Woodbridge Press Publishing Company
Post Office Box 6189
Santa Barbara, California 93111

Published simultaneously in the United States and Canada

Printed in the United States of America

Library of Congress Cataloging in Publication Data

Lawrence, Ronald Melvin, 1926–
  Pain relief with osteomassage.

  1. Pain—Treatment. 2. Massage. 3. Bones. I. Rosen-
berg, Stanley. II. Title.
RB127.L34 1982   615.8'22   82-13451
ISBN 0-912800-27-5

Pain Relief
with
Osteomassage

A simple yet effective treatment for many common pain problems, a treatment which under the guidance of a qualified health practitioner, can be self-administered or performed by another person.

Remember, of course, that no diagnosis or treatment of any medical condition should be undertaken without the advice of a qualified health practitioner.

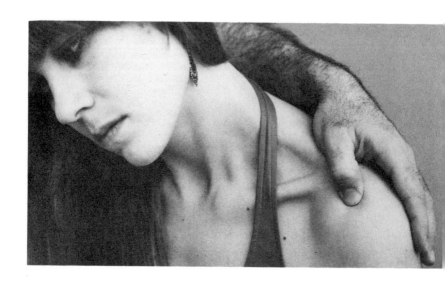

Contents

Osteomassage: an Introduction

Osteomassage is a technique for the relief of pain. It is an outgrowth from my work on the periosteum, the covering of the bone, beginning in 1973. I developed a technique, called *Osteopuncture*, for stimulation of the periosteum to treat painful disorders. Osteopuncture has been used to treat thousands of patients to date, not only by myself but by numerous physicians throughout the world.

Unlike *Osteomassage*, which *requires only the use of the fingertips*, Osteopuncture is performed by inserting small needles into the covering of the bone at various points throughout the body. After many studies, both in animals and in humans, this technique was found to be extremely effective in the treatment of pain problems. This work has been verified in many other laboratories and by other scientists not only in the United States of America but throughout the world. It is estimated that more than one hundred thousand patients have been treated with this technique since its discovery. I have personally treated more than six thousand patients in my North Hollywood, California, office. More than one thousand physicians have learned the technique and most of these doctors are applying it in their daily practice.

9

Osteomassage was developed as a logical extension of Osteopuncture techniques for stimulating the covering of the bone, *by using only the fingertips.* The methods described in this book have been carefully developed in practice. You will also find some information on the research done to explain why these techniques work.

However, it can be briefly stated that the periosteum (the thin covering of the surface of the bone) has a rich nerve and blood supply. Stimulation of this covering causes significant changes in the area treated by Osteomassage. These changes include an increase of the blood flow in the area and frequently result in the relief of pain. I think that you will find these methods to be most helpful, especially if pain problems have not responded to other forms of treatment.

PLEASE NOTE: *It is important to stress the fact that no one should attempt to treat a painful condition unless it has been adequately diagnosed by a physician or other qualified health practitioner and the treatment is undertaken with his approval. Pain is a warning signal which must be respected. Pain tells you that something may be seriously wrong and directs you to find the cause and to remedy the situation as quickly as possible.*

The Osteomassage techniques described in this book are especially useful in the treatment of chronic pain problems such as recurrent low back pain, knee pain, neck pain and other such pains. These recurrent pains are frequently secondary to conditions such as arthritis, slow-healing ligament injury, or persistent muscle problems.

Acute pain problems, such as those caused by sprain or athletic injuries, also respond very well to Osteomassage.

Overuse syndromes, arthritis, and recurrent headaches, are also especially responsive to this form of therapy.

Headaches are a special form of pain and like other painful conditions should be carefully investigated. A headache can be associated with a brain tumor or some other internal problem. Once a diagnosis is made, with the approval of the physician these Osteomassage methods may be helpful in obtaining relief from pain.

Throughout the book suggestions for the use of a particular technique will be given along with indications of the conditions that may be best treated by the technique. Please pay special attention to these indications for treatment of a particular area.

There are approximately 120 "*Osteopoints*" in the body. I will discuss only those that are important for the treatment of common pain problems. Should you have any questions regarding the techniques described in this book please feel free to write to me at the address given at the back of the book.

"Osteo-" comes from the Greek word for bone, *osteon*. "Massage" comes from the French word *masser* which means to knead or rub a part of the body, usually with the hands; or, typically in Osteomassage, a finger or thumb.

We recommend two to five minutes of massage over a bony area indicated as an "Osteopoint," rather than steady downward pressure. It is preferable to make small circular motions. These small motions can frequently stimulate a wider area of the periosteum.

One can use the eraser end of a pencil, or any soft object of about the same size, to exert pressure over the points we describe. Generally, though, we prefer to use finger pressure. It is safer and easier. However, when an individual tries to treat himself it may be difficult to maintain finger pressure long enough to complete the treatment. At such times a pencil with an eraser or a similar object can be helpful.

It is not necessary to use a lubricant but it will help you in making the small circular or massaging motions more effectively—unless you use too much. I recommend mineral oil as a lubricant, because it is so inexpensive and easy to obtain. However, any type of lubricant can be used and many are available in both drug stores and health food stores. The choice of lubricant is not as important as the technique with which you stimulate the bony areas. To remove mineral oil use rubbing alcohol. The use of any type of lubricant or rubbing alcohol is not recommended if the area involved has a cut or abrasion or is injured in some other way. In such cases wait until the injury has healed before attempting to treat the area.

The forefinger of the dominant hand (typically the right hand) usually can apply the type of pressure necessary for Osteomassage treatment. For some people the middle finger is more easily used. For others the thumb is the ideal digit because greater pressure can be administered. Whichever finger is used you will find that as you become familiar with the techniques you will have certain preferences based on the amount of pressure you can bring to bear against the bone and how comfortable you personally feel in using a particular digit.

In the photographs which illustrate the techniques you will note that sometimes the forefinger is used and sometimes the thumb. In such cases you can make your own choice as to which digit to use.

Again, remember that small circular massage movements are used at each designated site for about two to five minutes. Judge the length of treatment by the comfort of the patient. Do not cause discomfort in the bony area as you perform the massage. And, of course, in treating yourself, you will likewise be careful not to cause too much pain.

A dull, aching sensation, generated by either pressure or massage, is common and frequently indicates that the treatment is going to be effective. However any sharp or otherwise unacceptable pain means that you are over-stimulating the area. You would no doubt get results from such a treatment but it is not wise to subject yourself or a friend to such discomfort.

With older patients and children, whose skin is more easily injured, be exceptionally careful. Too much pressure may cause a breaking of small blood vessels in the skin, resulting in "black-and-blue" marks. It is better to under-treat than to overtreat.

Remember also that Osteomassage techniques are never

a cure. They are only simple techniques to diminish or alleviate common pain problems. Treatment of the actual cause of the pain as well as approval of the use of Osteomassage for the relief of pain, must be sought from a physician or other qualified health practitioner.

Ronald M. Lawrence, M.D.
North Hollywood, California

Fundamentals of
Osteomassage Treatment

Position of the Person To Be Treated

Preferably the person being treated should be lying down, comfortable and relaxed, in as natural a position as possible. If a subject is sitting up, he should be comfortable, preferably resting against some object so that he can more easily relax. Relaxation is most important. No treatment should be performed when the subject is tense or when the muscles are tight because the person is in an uncomfortable position. If you are treating yourself you also should be lying down, or in as comfortable a position as possible.

Digital Pressure

The amount of pressure you apply depends on the physique and the condition of the treated person. As we stated earlier, old or very young persons require special care. It is always best to start with light pressure, then gradually increase the pressure as you learn how the individual accepts the treatment and what occurs after light pressure techniques.

Generally you should use light pressure:

1. When you treat a person for the first time, even yourself.

2. When the pain is acute or of recent onset such as some athletic injuries. Always be certain that there are no underlying fractures of the bone.

3. Where there is swelling or puffiness around the bony area.

4. When there are medical complications, such as heart trouble, lung disease, high blood pressure or muscle wasting.

5. When the subject is obviously old with delicate bone structure. Heavy pressure on an individual who is old could conceivably cause not only bruising but also a bone fracture in certain areas and extra care must be taken.

6. When treating a young person whose skin is still delicate or who might not be cooperative or who does not understand the techniques being used. Time must be taken to explain the techniques to a child. We find that this usually results in cooperation. Such cooperation is important to effective treatment.

Harder pressure can be applied:

1. To individuals who have a chronic pain problem.

2. To persons who exhibit good bony structure.

3. To persons who have had at least one previous treatment.

Again, *chronic* problems respond to heavier pressure than do acute problems. The more *acute* the pain problem the less pressure is needed to control it.

Osteomassage Techniques

Massage should consist of small circular movements at a rate of about two to three cycles per second.

If pressure is being applied it is better to apply it directly downward against the surface of the bone, if at all possible, rather than at an angle to the bone.

You can massage two areas simultaneously, using both hands, but since the technique requires a great deal of energy, it is usually better to use one hand. If you do use two hands over two different areas at the same time you must coordinate your movements.

Again, it is most important to direct the pressure against the bony point only. In the photographs which follow you can study the position of the finger. You should always feel the bone immediately beneath the finger. If the bony surface is large start the massage or pressure techniques from the central portion of the bone.

Frequently throughout this book we use the term Osteopressure, either alone or along with the term Osteomassage. Osteopressure is the same as Osteomassage except that the small circular movements of stimulus on the Osteopoints are not used. Rather, a steady pressure (but not so hard as to cause discomfort) is applied to the Osteopoint. This pressure can last from a few seconds to several minutes or more.

Frequency of Treatment

Treatments can be given daily or even two or three times daily, depending upon the patient's response. However, when treating for the first time, we recommend giving only a single treatment per day. As you can study the reaction of the person or yourself you can increase the frequency of treatments to two or three times per day if necessary.

If you plan to treat several areas of the body at one time, it is best to start with only one area on the first day, then add an area each day as desired.

If you are treating a person with arthritis which involves many joints, you may start with only one or two, then gradually increase the number. You may eventually be able to treat all the joints involved at one time, if you have enough time and if the person is not too tired by the treatment. This may require as much as one hour of treatment. I would suggest not continuing the treatments beyond one hour since the person will probably become fatigued and the stimulation may be too much for such an extended time.

Other Treatment Information

1. The person who is treating should make sure that his hands are clean and warm. Never exert downward pressure against the bone with long fingernails since this may cut the skin.

2. The areas being treated should be kept warm but not uncomfortably so. If you are treating only one part of the body try to cover other parts of the body to keep them warm, exposing only the area being treated.

3. It is usually best not to treat a person right after he has eaten a heavy meal.

4. Avoid treating a person with an injured skin surface, from a cut, abrasion, contusion (black-and-blue-mark), or other cause. If you are advised by a physician to treat over such an area, cover it with a piece of sterile gauze and use the Osteomassage technique very gently.

5. Always terminate treatment if the patient's symptoms become worse or if the person becomes uncomfortable. Never urge a person to continue a treatment if he does not want to. This applies to yourself as well. If you feel uncomfortable or if any unusual sensations develop, stop the treatment and take a rest. If you try to do it again and the discomfort or sensations recur, discontinue the treatment until a later date and seek further advice from your physician.

Diet Suggestions

Although this book does not deal directly with diet I do wish to mention the relationship between diet and pain problems. I have found from experience that patients who eat a large amount of sugar will experience more pain. Such persons should reduce sugar intake. Sugar obtained from fruit is helpful, but refined carbohydrate, such as contained in candy, ice cream or table sugar, is to be avoided.

Sugar does not appear to increase the pain of an acute problem, such as an athletic injury but it often aggravates chronic pain. This is especially true concerning arthritis.

Alcoholic beverages are not recommended. Alcohol usually will make a pain much worse. Sometimes small amounts of alcohol, which relax a patient, seem to be helpful, but alcohol is generally to be avoided, especially by persons with chronic pain problems.

Fried or fatty foods can aggravate chronic pain. The effects of such foods will not be felt for forty-five minutes to one hour after ingestion.

Healthful, natural foods, such as fruits, vegetables, some kinds of nuts (and if meat is used—fresh meat, especially poultry or fish) are products that can be helpful to patients with chronic pain problems.

I recommend that persons who suffer from chronic pain study some of the numerous books available concerning diet and nutrition and develop a dietary program that promotes optimum health and well-being.

Guide to Treatments: How To Use This Book

This book is designed in a simple fashion so that under the guidance of a qualified health practitioner you can quickly find and use the information you need. Body areas affected by pain are listed alphabetically, starting with ankle pain and concluding with wrist pain. The general techniques of Osteomassage have clearly been described. The following photographs will illustrate the area or areas to be treated, with black dots showing where you can locate the underlying bone. Then the area is shown with a thumb or finger in position to apply Osteomassage.

Some indications for the treatment, which usually include treatment of both acute and chronic pain, will be listed in association with the photographs. Remember, it is important to apply the pressure only to the bony areas. Unless you can feel the bone do not administer the treatment.

In some of the areas we recommend that several Osteopoints be used. These points can be treated simultaneously or in a sequential fashion. It is not always necessary to treat every designated point in an involved area but usually it is more effective to do so. Sometimes a person will have more pain when you treat one particular spot so it may be advisable to change to another Osteopoint in the same general area.

Read carefully the section by Stanley Rosenberg, "Osteomassage as Practiced in Europe," which follows this Guide to Treatments.

Again, if you have any questions, please write to me at the address listed at the back of this book.

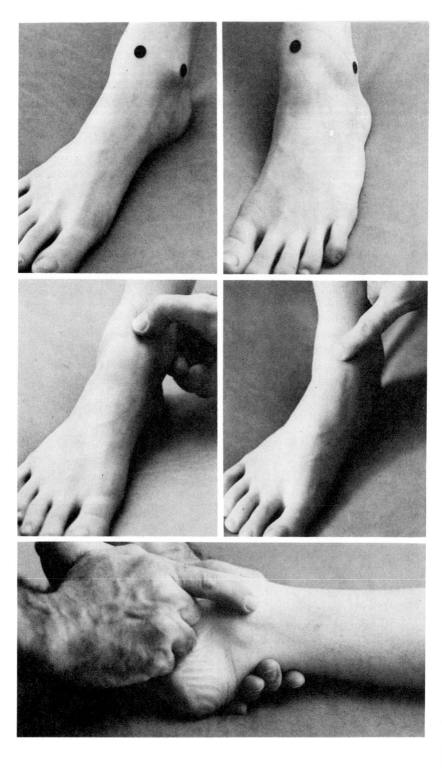

Ankle

Acute Pain

Sprain of the outside or the inside of the ankle.
Pain following excessive use of the ankle such as in running
or jogging a long distance.

Chronic Pain

Arthritis of the ankle joint, either degenerative arthritis
(osteoarthritis) or destructive arthritis (rheumatoid arthritis).

The treatment of degenerative arthritis, which is the
most common type, can be more extensive at first, more
pressure can be applied when beginning treatment, than is
the case with the destructive type of arthritis (rheumatoid
arthritis). When treating patients with destructive arthritis, great care should be taken, especially at the beginning. Such patients usually have delicate skin or skin which
is easily injured. Therefore, pressure must be carefully ex-
erted. A blend of Osteomassage and Osteopressure can frequently be very helpful in these conditions. We recommend
Osteopressure, applied for two minutes, and then a two-to-
five minute Osteomassage procedure.

Photographs A and B show the preferred Osteopoints.
Photograph C shows the thumb in position to apply
steady pressure or pressure with a circular motion. The
thumb can be used on any of the Osteopoints shown.
Photograph D illustrates use of the forefinger. Use the
digit you are most comfortable with or with which you can
apply the type of pressure desired.
Photograph E shows the ankle cradled with the left
hand, a useful technique. This sometimes achieves a
greater relaxation of the joint and the person will be more
comfortable during treatment.

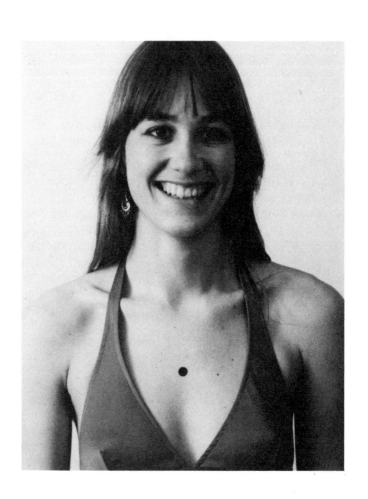

Chest

Acute Pain

Rib sprain, sprain of the ligaments which attach to the ribs.

Chronic Pain

Arthritis of the chest wall or front part of the chest.

When using the Osteopoint shown in the photograph, be very careful in applying pressure. If the patient finds it uncomfortable or if you find it uncomfortable, then it is better not to use this point too vigorously. In treating pain secondary to rib sprains (so-called "locked rib") it is sometimes better to work along the bony areas of the back until a tender spot or "trigger point" is located. Osteomassage at that point may be more effective in relieving pain.

Caution! Chest pain can be a sign of a "heart attack," and if especially severe or persistent, or if there is any indication whatever of heart involvement, a physician should be consulted—as indeed a qualified practitioner should be consulted for a diagnosis of any health problem.

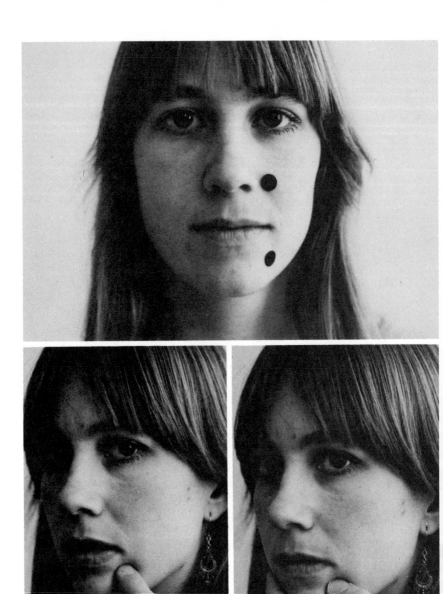

Chin

Acute Pain

Toothache involving the lower jaw.

Chronic or Recurrent Pain

"Facial tic" *(tic douloureux).*

Photographs A, B, C show the Osteopoints and alternative ways of applying Osteopressure. The upper point lies along the fold which runs from the side of the nose to the upper lip.

The upper point or the lower point may be used to treat the pain depending on the location of the "tic."

"Facial tic" is one of the most severe pains that a human being can have and instant success cannot be expected in many cases. A series of treatments may be necessary.

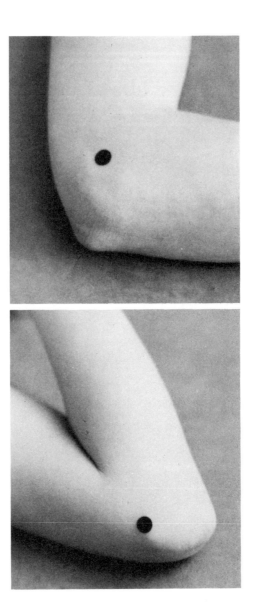

Elbow

Acute Pain

Elbow strain

Chronic or Recurrent Pain

Tennis elbow
Sprain of the major muscle *(pronator teres)* along the back
of the forearm.

A common painful condition for tennis players is "tennis
elbow." In addition to Osteotechniques, changing the
method of playing, such as correcting the backhand or
forehand strokes, must be considered. Sometimes a slight
change in the grip width of the racquet can be very helpful.

Both the inside and the outside parts of the elbow can be
involved. The respective Osteopoints are shown in *Photographs A and B*.

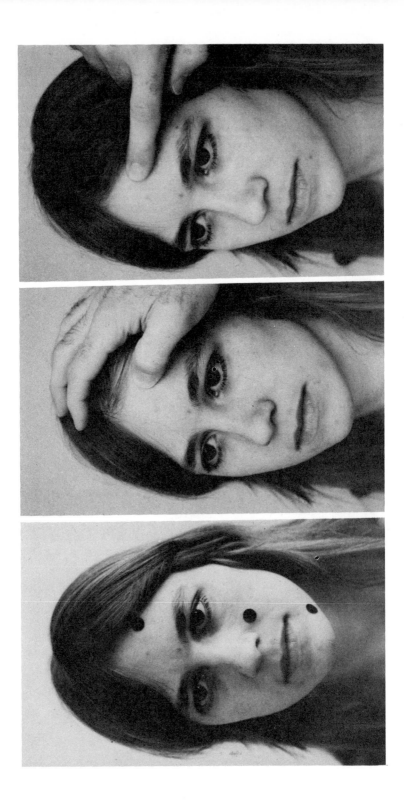

Face

(See also Chin, T.M. Joint, and Headaches)

Acute Pain

Sinusitis
Toothache
Headache

Chronic Pain

"Facial tic" *(tic douloureux).* (See this section.)
Sinusitis
Headaches

Photographs A, B, C show the Osteopoints and alternative Osteomassage positions.

The upper Osteopoint is helpful with frontal sinusitis and with headaches secondary to nervous tension. The middle Osteopoint is helpful with auxillary sinusitis and upper jaw toothache.

31

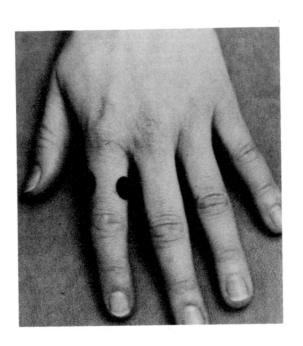

Finger

Acute Pain

Finger sprain, such as "baseball finger."

Chronic Pain

Degenerative arthritis (osteoarthritis)
Destructive arthritis (rheumatoid arthritis)

The photograph shows Osteopoints. Similar points can be used on any finger joint involved.

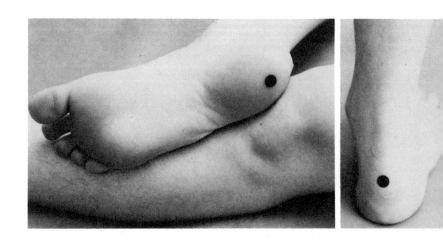

Heel

Acute Pain

Sprain of the ligament at the back of the heel
Pain associated with tight shoes

Chronic Pain

Arthritic pain
Heel spur pain

Proper footwear is important. Shoes should fit without too much restriction but neither should they be too loose. Heels that are too high can cause trouble. Sometimes a heel pad, available at most drug stores, can help.

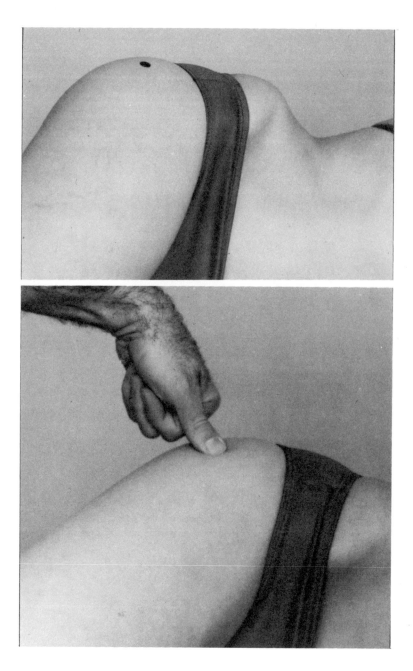

Hip

Acute pain, secondary to sprain, will often follow excessive running or stair climbing. In football injuries this is sometimes called a "pointer" chronic pain and may relate to both osteoarthritis or to rheumatoid arthritis (destructive arthritis).

If the pain is severe, especially in an older person, you may be dealing with bone fracture and X rays may be necessary before treatment. If it isn't a fracture you can usually safely use osteotechniques, guided by a qualified health practitioner. Sometimes a simple shoe pad or heel pad can be helpful.

The person is best treated if he is lying on his side. Sometimes a pillow placed between the thighs or legs may make it easier to feel the thigh bone.

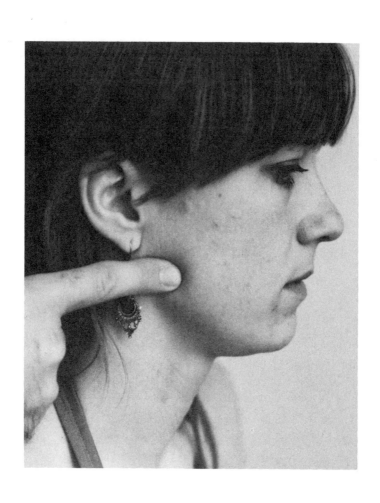

Jaw

(Angle of the lower jaw)

This point is especially useful in alleviating the pain of toothache in the lower jaw and; again, with the advice of a physician, for lockjaw. Lockjaw can develop after a lot of chewing or after "teeth grinding"—usually during the night. Both jaw angles can receive Osteomassage at the same time since this helps the involved side.

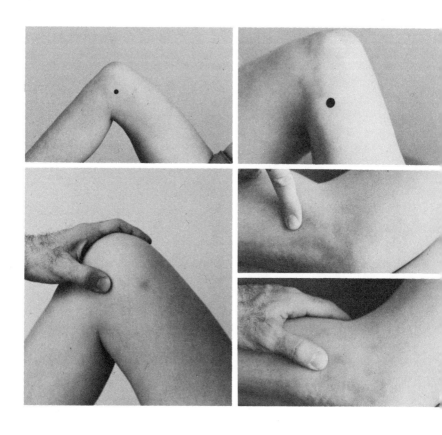

Knee

Outside knee pain can result from poor footwear, sprains and strains. You can feel the Osteopoint easily just below and to the side of the kneecap, the spot is about the size of a small coin.

Inside knee pain can result from poor footwear, splayfoot (a condition in which the toes point more outward than they should), arthritis of all types, torn cartilage, sprains and strains. The Osteopoint can be felt immediately below and to the inside of the kneecap at the ridge where you can feel the knee bending. This is the Osteopoint most associated with arthritic pain.

Remember the importance of good shoes!

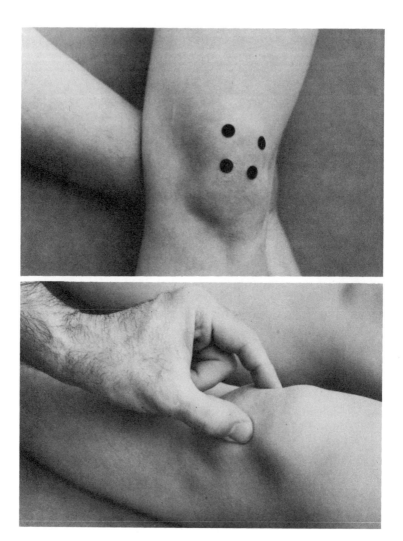

Kneecap

People often feel knee pain that is mainly around the kneecap. This type of pain may be caused by poor foot mechanics, which may be due to structural abnormalities ("fallen arches," for example), or poor footwear. It also can be due to all types of arthritis. All four Osteopoints can be used or only two of the four around the kneecap. Gently rocking the kneecap back and forth sometimes will aid in the treatment, but remember, "be gentle"!

Hip, knee, foot or ankle pain is sometimes relieved by treatment of all four areas shown. That is because these four areas are all intimately connected and related. Problems in one of the areas can involve another area or areas. The old song which alleges that the "foot bone is connected to the ankle bone, the ankle bone is connected to the knee bone" and so on, couldn't be more correct.

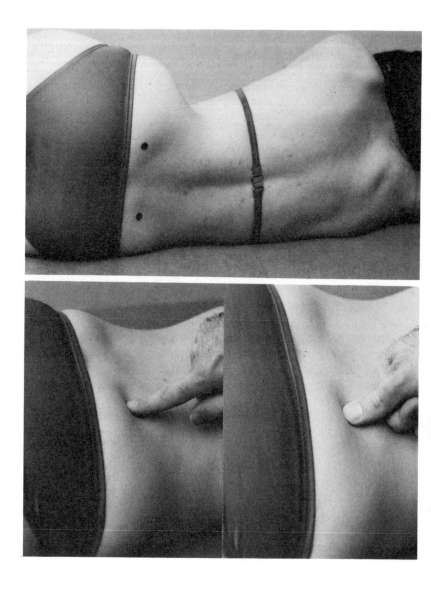

Lower Back

(Also see Upper and Middle Back)

Acute Pain

Back sprain or lumbago

Chronic Pain

Osteoarthritis (degenerative arthritis)
Rheumatoid arthritis (destructive arthritis)
"Slipped disc"

These Osteopoints can be felt at the areas where the "dimples" are located in the low back. They are about one to one and one-half inches from the spine. These Osteopoints work especially well. Combining the treatment with application of heat or cold is effective. Allow thirty minutes of rest after the Osteomassage or Osteopressure, if possible.

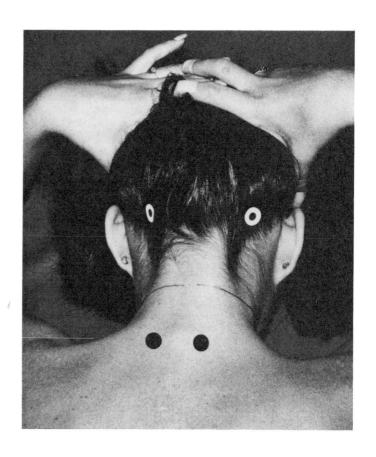

Neck

(Also see Headaches)

These Osteopoints, located where the skull joins the neck are useful in treating not only upper neck pain but also headaches which begin at or involve the back of the head. The muscles most affected by stress are attached to these Osteopoints.

Deep breathing of the patient while these Osteopoints are being treated (with the patient lying down), can also help to relax the neck muscles.

Neck

(Lower part—also see Shoulder)

If the main pain involves the lower neck, these Osteopoints are especially useful. They are located about one inch to the side of that part of the spine that "sticks out" where the neck joins the upper back.

In shoulder pain these Osteopoints may be very tender.

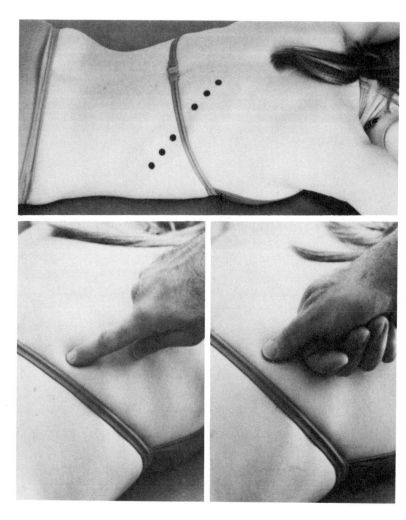

Rib

Although you can treat anywhere along the involved rib, sometimes one point is better than another. That is why we show so many Osteopoints along the rib line.

Caution! Do not rub these Osteopoints if there is rib fracture. If a broken rib is suspected you should not use any of the techniques because you could push the broken rib into the lung area and perhaps even cause a "collapsed lung."

Remember here as well as elsewhere, if you are in doubt, don't treat.

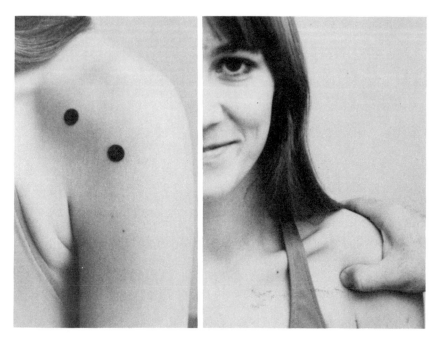

Shoulder

Acute Pain

Sprain of the ligaments or tendon
Bursitis, or acute inflammation of the joint sac

Chronic Pain

Secondary to either osteoarthritis or rheumatoid arthritis
Recurrent tendinitis
Recurrent bursitis

Osteotechniques can be supplemented with hot or cold packs to the affected part. In acute conditions, cold or ice packs are better; for chronic conditions heat may be better, moist heat particularly. Sometimes alternating hot and cold packs can be helpful. Remember also that motion in the shoulder joint is important and should be gently performed. If the person performs this motion "on his own" then you can assist. *Remember:* never move the part beyond the point that the shoulder begins to hurt. Never force the movement.

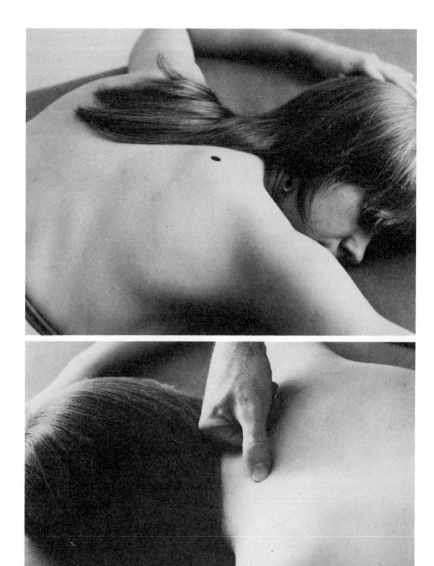

Shoulder Blade

The Osteopoint is located at the inner tip of the shoulder blade about two inches from the spine. It usually is a tender place even in normal conditions. It is a point where muscles from the neck, as well as shoulder muscles, insert. Many persons develop pain or ache here due to everyday tensions. Neck pain often accompanies the shoulder blade pain. Sometimes pain develops here due to poor posture or from sitting for long hours in a chair or in an upright (or "up tight") position. Pain here sometimes follows "whiplash" of neck and shoulders associated with automobile or other vehicular accidents.

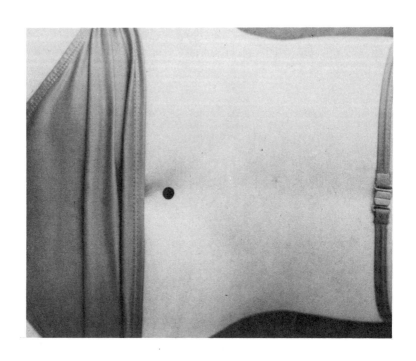

Tailbone

Pain in this location is sometimes called coccydynia. It may be caused by sitting on hard surfaces. It may occur after childbirth, especially if it was a difficult delivery or if baby's head was especially large. Such pain may also begin after a fall onto the area. In addition to Osteomassage, sitting on a pad or a "doughnut" type ring or other soft surfaces will help. Heat and ice, or both together may also help. Sitting in a tub of hot water is frequently helpful. You can feel the Osteopoint at the tip of the bone.

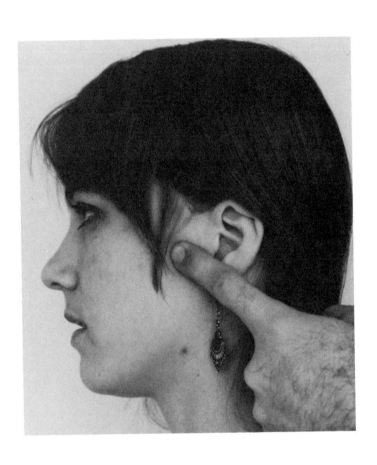

T.M. Joint

This is the so-called T.M. *(temporo-mandibular)* joint. Many people with dental problems may have pain here and of course they should also see a dentist. You can feel the joint when the person opens or closes the jaw. It is immediately in front of the ear.

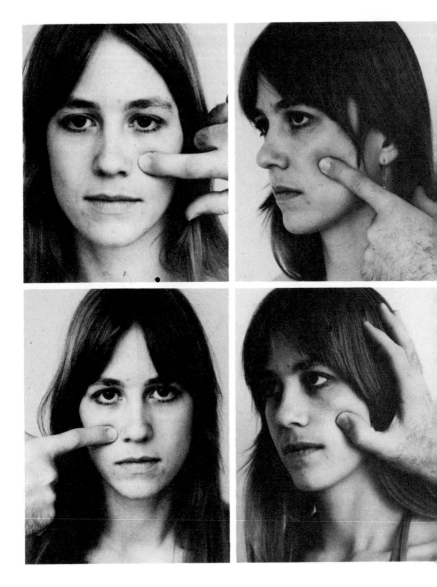

Toothache

(Also see Jaw and Face)

Toothache pain at this point can be relieved by pressing on the involved dental area. Again, a dentist should be consulted.

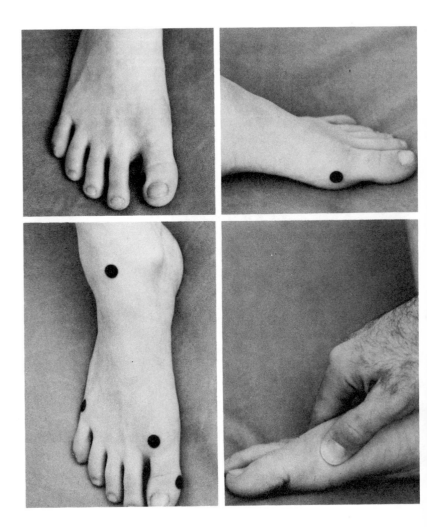

Toe

(Also see Heel)

The first photograph shows osteopoints at the so-called "bunion area," where bunions most frequently develop. Poorly fitting footwear is responsible for many of these problems. The patient should see a podiatrist (foot doctor). Bunions can also involve the little toe. Arthritis can involve any part of any of the toes. The Osteopoints are located on either side of the involved joint or joints.

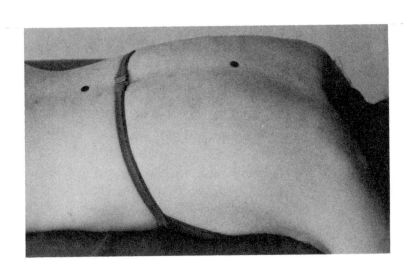

Upper and Middle Back

Osteopoints are located along the upper and middle spinal area. The bony protrusions all along the spine are each excellent Osteopoints. Just locate the area where the pain is and you can feel the bone at that location (the spinous process).

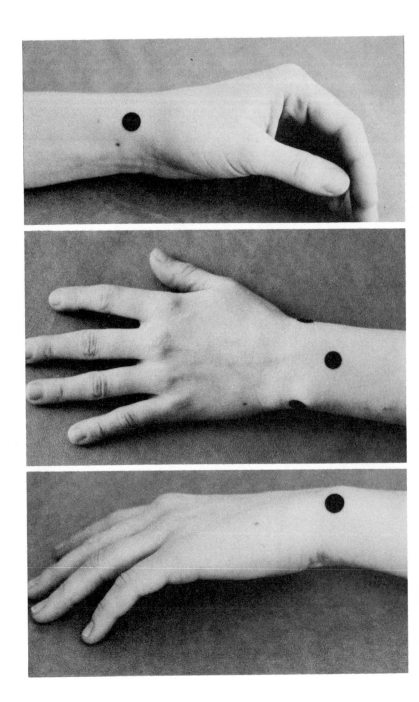

Wrist

Osteopoints at the wrist are on either side of the wrist and also at a point on the back of the wrist, between the side points. Wrist pain can be related to all types of arthritis, sprains and bursitis. In addition to Osteomassage and Osteopressure, a wrist elastic bandage or a wrist strap is often helpful, both of which can be purchased at a drug store.

Alternating hot and cold packs or soaks can also help to relieve the discomfort. Again, if you suspect a fracture avoid using Osteotechniques.

Stanley Rosenberg of Denmark has taken the basic principles of Osteopuncture and Osteomassage as I taught them to him several years ago and developed a European approach to Osteomassage. He and his colleagues have refined some of my methods and developed some new ones. This supplement to the book is included so that the reader may have a comprehensive understanding of some of the varied Osteomassage techniques available today in different parts of the world. The reader, in consultation with a physician, may elect to use methods described by Mr. Rosenberg or may modify those described by either him or me to create a comfortable blend of treatments. Both his techniques and mine are based on the principles discovered in Osteopuncture research. Both produce essentially similar results. The European method as described here by Mr. Rosenberg is taught in special classes. The American method, as I have described it in this book is somewhat easier to apply for the average person who does not attend a class or take other formal instruction. Both methods, used in cooperation with professional health practitioners, will open an exciting new pathway to health and happiness.

—Ronald M. Lawrence, M.D.

Osteomassage
as Practiced in Europe

By Stanley Rosenberg

Introduction

Osteomassage is a form of holistic healing that is effective on the physical, emotional, mental and spiritual levels. It is easy to learn. It is easy to do. It works because it is attuned to existing structures in the nervous system.

This direct stimulation of the nervous system by massage on the bony structure of the body has helped many people achieve better balance, increased flexibility, and greater clarity.

Osteopuncture, the foundational precursor of *Osteomassage*, first came into prominence in the United States. Dr. Lawrence and hundreds of physicians who studied with him have had extremely positive results with it in relieving pain. In more than one hundred thousand cases, without drugs or operations, they have helped an amazingly high percentage of patients to overcome pain. Their case histories serve to document the fact that Osteopuncture works.

In a more recent development, in Europe, we use Osteomassage as a technique to further the growth of personal awareness and extend states of consciousness in the pursuit of spiritual development. In order to enjoy our lives more fully and in order to survive, we need full use of our mental capacity, emotional sensitivity and physical well-being. Hundreds of people in several countries have attended short courses in Osteomassage to become more able to help themselves, to help people that they care about, or to learn its uses as a form of psychophysical therapy to help others in the community.

People attending Osteomassage courses in Europe have a variety of backgrounds. Some have professional training and practice in areas of traditional health care: for example, medical doctors, physiotherapists, and psychologists. Others have no previous experience with health care, healing or psychophysical therapy forms. In their occupations, they include real estate salesmen, bus drivers, students, housewives, school teachers, and others.

The professional people were generally surprised that Osteomassage was so effective, so simple and that it could be used in so many situations. The nonprofessionals found Osteomassage easy to learn and many reported satisfaction that they could use the techniques and get good results from what they learned in an intensive weekend course.

Osteomassage works because it stimulates a mechanism in the nervous system. Stimulation of the nervous system in the proper way produces specific, predictable, beneficial effects. Once you learn what that mechanism is and how to stimulate it, you will have a practical knowledge you can use to help other people.

One of the first things that people notice when they receive Osteomassage is a deep relaxation. Within a few minutes, they have a good feeling. Stress, anxiety, fear and guilt give way to a pleasant state of peace and harmony. After the treatment is over, people usually experience increased clarity and sense more energy.

In addition to the immediate effects, Osteomassage is

educational. It teaches the person how to relax in a way that he can use naturally in other situations.

People who have Osteomassage in a series of treatments once a week for several weeks, generally notice a dramatic rise in their ability to deal with and overcome problems in their life. They begin to do more of what they really want with their time. Emotionally, they experience joy and satisfaction more and more often.

Most of us walk around trying to solve our problems while operating at far less than our potential ability. Our capabilities are limited because of blockages caused by tensions.

Our lives are often filled with stress, worry, doubts, restlessness, emptiness, or loneliness. We are all too aware of the impact of international political crises, the gradual destruction of the life-supporting environment of our planet, rising prices and decreasing job-security, and occasional difficulties in family relationships and personal friendships.

To meet such challenges, we need all of our personal resources. The more balance we can achieve, the more effective we can become, the more we will be in a position to establish a higher quality of life for ourselves and for the people close to us.

More and more people are looking toward new methods, to holistic methods. People are more willing to take responsibility and do something to improve their own health— better diet, more exercise, meditation, massage, and so on.

Most of the drugs people take stimulate or depress the nervous system, repress emotional expression, or suppress certain states of mind. The pills—whether prescribed by a doctor or obtained illegally—affect the nervous system by speeding it up or slowing it down. While the drug is working, we are speeded up or slowed down regardless of changes in the real situation around us.

The body, however, has its own built-in mechanism for slowing down and speeding up. That mechanism is the autonomic part of the nervous system. When the autonomic nervous system operates properly, it is a reflection of our

real-life situation, and it provides us with the necessary
level of energy to be successful.

Osteomassage brings responsiveness and balance to the
autonomic nervous system so that we can function naturally, without drugs—in balance, in harmony, and with ful-
ler appreciation of our human potential.

Let us first take a look at the autonomic nervous system
and see how it functions to regulate the body and how it
relates to mental and emotional states. In Osteomassage
courses in Europe, even people with no previous knowledge of anatomy had no trouble in learning the techniques
because the underlying principles were presented clearly,
in simple terms. They gained confidence based on their
understanding and could then interpret the various effects
they produced in giving Osteomassage to someone else.

After we have our basic understanding of the autonomic
nervous system, then we will go step-by-step into the de-
tails of an effective Osteomassage technique and learn how
to do it.

How Osteomassage Works

When we give Osteomassage to someone, we apply light
pressure to various areas of the bony structure of the body.
To be more precise, we pressurize a thin, living membrane
which surrounds the hard, bony mineral deposits. That
membrane is called the periosteum. The periosteal membrane contains many blood vessels and is rich in nerve endings.

We can often, literally "feel it in our bones." This is because these nerve endings on the periosteum are very sensitive. They pick up information not only about touch, but
also heat, cold, and sound. Once these various kinds of
stimuli are picked up by the nerve endings on the periosteum, they are transformed into pulses. These pulses carry
the information farther along different pathways to two
destinations in the nervous systems.

One pathway moves the signal to the spine, up the spinal cord, to the brain stem, into the thalamus (a kind of "switchboard" more or less in the center of the brain), and out to the cerebral cortex. The cerebral cortex is the outer layer of the brain. We can be conscious of signals which reach the cerebral cortex. That is why, when something or someone touches us on the bones, we can "know" where it is happening. If signals from the nervous system reach areas of the brain other than the cerebral cortex, or other nerve centers in the other parts of the body, we do not "know" about them. They are below the level of consciousness.

The second pathway from the periosteum reaches certain of these other nerve centers below the level of consciousness. Even though we don't know that the information is reaching these centers and even though we don't choose to do anything voluntarily, stimulation of these nerve centers produces strong, specific effects on the body.

These other nerve centers, which we can stimulate by pressure on the periosteum are part of what is called "the sympathetic division of the autonomic nervous system." It may be worthwhile here to discuss the various functions of the "autonomic nervous system," especially the "sympathetic division."

Although the words themselves ("sympathetic division of the autonomic nervous system") may seem like Greek to some, the functions they stimulate can at times, unfortunately, be all too familiar to most of us: poor circulation, high blood pressure, faulty digestion, loss of appetite or overeating, fast pulse, shallow breathing, irregular heartbeat, cold hands and feet, pale complexion, tight muscles, neck pain, hormone imbalance, rectal pain, eye troubles, emotional instability, insomnia, mental confusion, dry throat, and so on. If any of these symptoms trouble you or people that you care about, you may find that Osteomassage can help.

Most of the complaints that take people to the doctor for prescriptions or operations come from improper balance in the activity of the autonomic nervous system. Drugs often have undesirable side-effects and surgical operations are rarely reversable. It would be nice to have an alternative method that could be used in some of these instances.

The autonomic nervous system itself consists of two parts: the sympathetic division and the parasympathetic division. Increased energy in the nerves of the sympathetic division causes tension in the body, but increasing activity of the parasympathetic division brings about relaxation. Too much sympathetic stimulation can make us like an overwound watch spring. Too much flow in the parasympathetic can leave us a will-less blob, like a wet dish towel.

The words, "sympathetic" and "parasympathetic" do indeed come from the Greek. The prefix, *sym*, means to be with something (as in symphony, symbiosis, etc.). The word *"pathos"* may mean suffering or feeling. "Sympathetic" means to agree in feeling, or to suffer when another suffers. If we see someone else in pain, we don't have to "think" about it or "do" anything—the experience has already manifested in us and there is a response in our sympathetic nervous system, subconsciously and immediately. The prefix *para*, in some cases, means "beyond." So, parasympathetic means beyond suffering or feeling with someone else.

If we are suffering, we want to change what is happening or to get away. The sympathetic nervous system is associated with the "fight or flight" reaction—anger and fear. We perceive something that we don't want. However, the parasympathetic nervous system is activated from satisfaction, joy, sharing with others the positive things. In states of relaxation the body energy is focused on digesting and rebuilding the body tissues.

Last spring I saw a pony eating grass in a field. Suddenly a car came by and the driver sounded the horn. The horse was startled and started to run in the opposite direction. He was so angry or afraid he galloped away at top speed. He ran two or three hundred yards, stopped, looked around, and then put his head down and started to graze again.

THE NEW YORKER

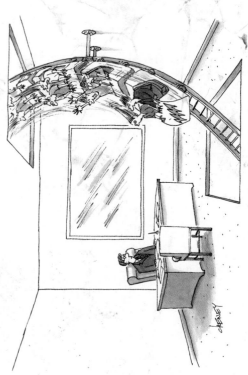

"This part of the ride always creeps me out."

When he was surprised by the sound of the horn, he had a strong flow of energy in the sympathetic nervous system. In an instant, his body was ready for strong physical action. Part of that energy was used up in the run. Now that he was farther away from the car and it was not so dangerous, he was able to relax. Energy increased in the parasympathetic nervous system and he returned to his pleasurable pastime of "eating like a horse."

If the horse responds to a real threat to his well-being, "fight or flight" is a good way of increasing his chances for survival. A horse suddenly seeing a rattlesnake will rear up, turn, and get away as fast as he can.

Sometimes a horse (especially if he is high-strung, or has been inquartered in a stable all winter) might react to something as if it were a threat; when, in fact, he is perfectly safe. Sometimes a horse will react to a shadow, or a puddle of water. That kind of behavior is considered neurotic— there is a mismatch between the interpretation of a situation as dangerous and the reality of a situation which is perfectly safe.

As people, we respond not only to physical reality, but also to our thoughts, memories, plans, symbols, emotions, etc. We respond fully to these nonphysical events as if they were physically dangerous, or physically nonthreatening: with a sympathetic or a parasympathetic response. Just look at how emotional we can get watching a football game or a television program or reading a newspaper.

As people, we can also react with fear to the sympathetic responses of our own nervous system. The original responses might have been caused by something else. Someone might be in a stress situation and notice his heart beating faster. This might make him afraid that there was something wrong with his heart. This fear would make his heart beat still faster. This could make him even more afraid. It is a vicious circle. It happens to a lot of people.

Much disease and tension is caused by fear arising from the activity of the sympathetic nervous system. In reality, our fear can make us pretty sick without our realizing it.

Probably half to one third of our stress-related illnesses
(and doctors list heart disease, cancer, and arthritis as diseases which occur often in people with anxiety) could be
prevented or cured if we could establish a more natural
movement of energy from the sympathetic and the
parasympathetic division of the nervous system. Just as in
the story of the horse in the field, when there is a real
danger we could be able to react fully and when there is no
longer any difficulty we should be able to let go and relax
fully.

Let us look in detail at these paths of expression when
we stimulate the sympathetic nervous system. What happens in the body when we perceive a dangerous or negative
situation? In a case of anxiety, we are stimulated but do not
act by fighting or running, and we do not relax again. What
happens to the body if the sympathetic nervous system is
excited over a long period of time?

In danger (anger or fear), a whole series of changes can
occur in the body. Essentially, we refocus the bodily resources from digestion and rebuilding to a full mobilization
of the muscles to be ready to fight or to run. The muscles
are ready to react strongly over an extended period of
time. Blood that had been used to digest food in the
stomach and intestines is now redirected to provide for the
muscles which will move the body.

One or more of the following things will happen as we
increase activity in the sympathetic division of the autonomic nervous system. Often, the muscles tighten. One
muscle pulls against the other. The body is ready to spring
in any direction. The increased tension will allow for
strong, quick, explosive movements. However, prolonged
muscle tension creates unnecessary strain in the body. We
sometimes notice that someone is "up tight" when the tension is general.

At other times, the muscle cramping is more localized.
We sometimes find that "he gives me a pain in the neck";
or, inelegantly, "he gives me a pain in the ass." (In the
latter case, "a backache" might be a less vigorous form of

expression, but more commonly the physical result of tense situations.) Tensions may be more on the right side of the body, or more on the left side. This is why some people have a "short" leg, or one shoulder that is "higher" than the other. Chronic tension can pull one of the vertebrae out of shape leading to backache or contributing to a "slipped" or ruptured disk.

With this increase of activity in the sympathetic nervous system, the muscles need the extra blood and oxygen so that they can work and also to carry away the by-products of their work. Thus, the heart starts to beat more rapidly. The breathing quickens. The blood pressure goes up. If we don't use the muscles and don't relax, then the breathing might remain quick, but we breath in a shallow way to keep from being flooded with too much oxygen. The high blood pressure comes about in part because of a constriction of the blood vessels. Cheeks of the face, once rosy pink, can turn pale and wan. There might also be increased irritability, lack of emotional balance, oversensitivity to sounds, lower threshold of pain, etc.

Coming back to the muscles, to get rid of the heat that we can expect from the violent actions of fighting or running, the "air conditioners" get turned on. The body begins to sweat. As the sweat on the surface of the skin dries, the evaporation causes cooling. We often say that someone who is angry is "hot under the collar." Sometimes, we will tell them to "cool it." If the coolers are on and we do not produce extra heat in the muscles, the body temperature falls below normal. Some people feel cool over their whole body. Others have cold hands, or cold, clammy feet. Indeed, we say that someone who is afraid has "cold feet," meaning that he will not face something.

While it is preparing the muscles, the sympathetic response of the nervous system also curtails the level of activity in the digestion of food. We may experience a loss of appetite or a lack of interest in food. Sometimes we find that the food seems to have lost its taste. For some people, the mouth or the throat gets dry. In order to make it more difficult to put food into the stomach, the body will stop the flow of saliva. Thus we have less interest in food, or we taste the food less, or we may develop a nervous cough from the dry throat.

Sometimes the food which is already in the stomach gets stopped from going further. In extreme cases, we may feel sick, queezy in our stomach, or we may feel nauseous. We may throw up if the shock is too great. In a mild anxiety, the food simply stops longer in the stomach than necessary and stomach acids may give us heart burn; or, for some people, after a period of time the situation can lead to an ulcer.

In other cases, the intestines will stop moving the food along. The rhythmic, fluid movement of the muscles of the intestines is called peristalsis. If the peristalsis stops, the food stops moving in the intestines. This is an advantage in a dangerous situation. Then we can direct more energy to other muscles. But if a temporary slowdown or stoppage of the peristalsis lasts too long, we get constipation. In some cases, the bacteria in the intestines will cause putrefaction. Poisonous by-products of this process enter the blood and among other things can cause migraine headaches. In extreme cases, the body doesn't stop the food for later digestion, it involuntarily empties the intestinal tract—now. Then everything is ready for fight or flight.

Also, we often observe a change in sexual functioning. If we are in balance, when there is an appropriate occasion for sexual activity, our body is aroused and we perform normally. The "appropriate occasion" has a lot to do with biological rhythms—for example, the season of the year, the time of the month for the woman, the social situation, the nature of the relationship, and so on. But when we start to get out of balance in the autonomic nervous system, one of two things starts to happen: 1. We start to get overactive, obsessively interested in sex; or, 2. we lose interest and cannot perform satisfactorily. So, in cases of imbalance, we get too much or too little sexual activity.

Many people have problems in marriage. If a partner is under stress one may feel pushed into more sex than is desired, or may find that the partner becomes cold and unresponsive. The sexual impulse may come at inappropriate times, or in situations which cause complications.

If after a stressful situation, we could relax, most of the problem physical symptoms would disappear. We would be in good health. We would enjoy ourselves more. The sympathetic nervous system controls these many and varied functions in the body. In a natural state, when men had a very hard existence, the autonomic nervous system allowed him to survive because the sympathetic nervous system mobilized his activities in the face of threat to life and limb. The parasympathetic response then relaxed him when danger was past. Those who managed their energy survived.

Certainly, in the mildly negative or stressful situations of everyday life, not all of these symptoms appear at the same time. If they did, we would not survive very long. Everyone is different and so the overactivity of the sympathetic nervous system will produce different effects. Part of the difference is our individual heredity, the genetic structure we inherited from our parents. Part of it is culture we grew up in. In some families, it is acceptable to get angry and blow off steam, while in other families, anger or fear is repressed, forcing the energy into other channels.

In a natural situation after a danger is passed, the parasympathetic nervous system in a well-balanced person will produce a change to relax the muscles, slow the heart and breathing, restore the digestion, and permit a harmonious sexual activity. There is return to a quiet, peaceful state of mind, body and emotions. But often, we do not get a chance to rest and balance out. We await another unpleasant encounter at work, we are afraid to go certain places alone at night, we worry about the future of our children, we see the flow of seemingly insoluble world problems on television news, we race from one place to another without time to do all that we want or what others expect from us.

We have found instead that we can do certain things to

ourselves which force the body to give up the overactivity of the sympathetic nervous system. But in all too many cases, we pay dearly in terms of health. Overeating, tranquilizing drugs, alcohol, and cigarettes are all things that we put into the body to suppress the sympathetic nervous system. All of these, continued over a long period of time produce unhealthy effects.

If we could only find a way to restore the function of our parasympathetic nervous system! If we could only find a way to make both the sympathetic and the parasympathetic nervous system more responsive to our moment-to-moment needs!

Osteomassage provides just such a way of retraining the autonomic nervous system to respond naturally. (It deconditions undesirable patterns of blockage through an effect which is called hyperstimulation analgesia. Hyperstimulation analgesia essentially erases patterns of memory of pain lodged in the thalamus, the "switchboard" of the brain.)

Often during or after Osteomassage you will hear a rumbling or gurgling sound in the stomach or abdomen, a sign that the peristalsis is going again, that the food is moving along in the intestinal tract.

The muscles relax.

Saliva starts to come into the mouth again, and often you will notice the person swallowing.

The heartbeat slows and the breathing slows and becomes deeper in character. On occasion, people will sigh with relief.

The lens of the eye changes shape, irrigation increases in the eyes and you will often notice tears (pleasant "tears of joy") run out of the corner of the eye.

There can also come a flow of renewed energy in the sexual parts of the body. (One of the positive things noticed by several people who have received Osteomassage is that they have developed a more responsive, satisfying sexual experience.)

In conclusion, we see that a great many seemingly different kinds of problems and diseases have a common cause in the nervous system. The techniques of Osteomassage can help many people with such a variety of problems because it restores a natural movement between the two divisions of the autonomic nervous system.

Much of the drug therapy developed over the last thirty years works to increase or decrease activity in the sympathetic or parasympathetic divisions of the autonomic nervous system. Many drugs have been found to produce harmful side effects. If a person is suffering in one state, the drugs can put him into another state, but they do not make him responsive in a natural way.

My brother told me a story about a young mountain climber who died of overexposure while his friends under the same circumstances survived. He had been taking drugs to manage high blood pressure. The drugs suppressed the activity of his sympathetic nervous system. The shock of cold weather and hard work would normally excite a person's sympathetic nervous system to mobilize his strength to be able to survive. For the others not on the drugs, this happened. For the unfortunate climber, his system, depressed by the drugs, could not respond to the new situations. He died.

Holistic healing seeks ways to restore our natural mechanisms of balance and free us from dependence on unnatural uppers or downers.

Osteomassage: How To Do It

As we said earlier, when we massage the bones, we stimulate the nerve endings on the periosteum, or the thin membrane covering the bones. Some of these nerve endings connect to centers in the sympathetic nervous system.

In Europe, we work with Osteomassage using a technique which gently stimulates the sympathetic nervous system. Within a short period of time after the stimulation of the sympathetic nervous system, the body recognizes that this sign of "danger" is gone. Energy then flows in the parasympathetic nervous system and brings with it a wave of relaxation. Repeating this process several times, each wave of activity in the parasympathetic nervous system takes the person deeper and deeper into a state of relaxation.

When Dr. Lawrence visited us in Copenhagen, he gave us a key in refining this process. The body has a response that you can feel with your fingertips telling you when the parasympathetic response has taken over. You can come to feel the pulse of the blood vessels of the periosteum when the parasympathetic response starts. This gives you a natural feedback system. Timing your movements in the massage to these effects produced in the nervous system of the person you are working with makes this special Osteomassage technique quite effective.

In terms of the healing, we use three words to describe the different parts of the technique. At the start, when we massage the bone, we *stimulate* the nervous system. Then, we wait while the sympathetic nervous system responds. This middle period we call the *release*. Then, at the end, just when we sense the feedback mechanism telling us that the parasympathetic system has responded, we call this, the *clearance*.

We work essentially with the system of Osteopoints, especially in our beginning courses. The method is simple to learn.

We use the middle finger, the long finger of the hand, which we feel most comfortable working with. This finger is especially sensitive, and because of the construction of the nerves of the hands and arms, sensing with this finger while we give the massage helps us, ourselves, to relax.

To use the special Osteomassage technique, place the middle finger lightly on one of the Osteopoints. Remember, you don't have to press very hard. You are stimulating the nerve endings surrounding the bone. It is enough if you can just feel, slightly, the surface of the hard part of the bone. A light touch facilitates your sensing of the body's own feedback system.

You stimulate by making a single, circular motion with

your finger tip. The skin moves with you, as you make the small circle. The circle need be no more than one-fourth of an inch in diameter, because of the rich concentration of nerve endings on the periosteum. One circle is enough. You don't have to keep rubbing. You have thus finished the *stimulation.*

Then comes the period of *release.* You keep your finger still, touching lightly on the bone, in the same place where you finished your circular movement in the stimulation part of the stroke.

After a period of time that might last anywhere from two seconds up to a minute, you will feel a small pulse under your fingertip. This is the flow of blood into the periosteum telling you that there has been a *clearance,* a relaxation, a flow of energy in the parasympathetic nervous system. When you feel the blood pulse, the little blip, you lift your finger completely free of the other person's body. Then you put your finger done on another part of the same bone, or you can move to another Osteopoint.

We usually work a succession of such processes on the same Osteopoint. Actually, the body has a network of nerve endings over the entire periosteum. But when we talk of Osteopoints, we really mean an area on the periosteum which has a richer concentration of nerve endings than other areas of the periosteum. Also, the Osteopoints are fairly easy to reach in massage, lying near the skin and not hidden by heavy muscle tissue. In reality, we can work anywhere on the surface of any bone that we can reach fairly easily.

When you have finished one massage process, it is usually a good idea to repeat the process close to the preceding site. You need not go far away. A distance of one-eighth of an inch is enough to get a completely fresh response. So, put your finger down one-eighth of an inch from the site of the preceding maneuver. Make a single, small circle *(stimulate).* Wait *(release).* When you sense the pulse, lift your finger *(clearance).* Repeat this process again and again.

Trust to the simplicity of the technique. It is easy to do, requiring almost no physical effort. After you have practiced for a while, you will find that in anywhere from 5 to 20 minutes, you can take most people to a state of deeper relaxation than they have known from almost any other experience—to a "center" of peace, harmony and calmness.

In the beginning, we suggest that you work from five to ten minutes on an Osteopoint before you move on to another point.

Trust to the techniques we described here. If you have patience and wait for the pulse, you will get a good result.

More about Sensing the Pulse

To use the technique in the most effective way, it is important to learn to sense the pulse. Therefore, since you may be reading this book at home and certain questions may arise for some of you, we want to go into this part of the work in more detail.

Even if you massage the Osteopoints without paying any attention to the pulse, you will produce a beneficial result for the person that you are working on. The reason we teach people to look for the pulse—and time the massage strokes to the "blip" on the periosteum is to make you more effective, to allow you to work deeper in less time.

It also will help you relax yourself, to relax more deeply while giving the massage. We observe an interesting phenomenon. When you give Osteomassage to others, you can often reach a state of superconsciousness yourselves. You can feel very awake and at the same time sense a deep relaxation in your own mind and body. That is one of the joys of working with Osteomassage.

Most people will feel the pulse under their fingertips within a few practice strokes. It is not an earth-shaking volcano. If your touch is light, you will sense it, even though it is of less intensity than feeling the arterial pulse on someone's wrist.

Once you start to recognize what the pulse feels like to

you, you will start to notice that it takes a different length of time for the pulse to come back from one stroke to the next. One might be very quick. Another might take a long time. The reason for this has to do with the nervous pathway from the periosteum to the cerebral cortex on the surface of the brain. If the specific nerve endings that you touch have never been shocked by a painful experience, the nervous impulse travels freely and quickly up to the cerebral cortex. The pulse under your finger comes back very quickly. If there has been a painful experience, it takes longer.

For example, if you fell down some stairs, or were hit by a stick, or hit yourself on the edge of a table, the nerves that carried that pain to the brain create a memory pattern in the thalamus. When we restimulate the nerves in the Osteomassage, it calls up a series of past experiences in a somewhat subconscious dream-like experience in the consciousness of the person receiving the massage. If there has been pain in the past this dream-like state of release goes on for a period of time, usually lasting some seconds. The activity in the thalamus produces an effect which is called hyperstimulation analgesia. Here is the best way to describe hyperstimulation analgesia: imagine that the nerve junctions in the thalamus are like the circuit breakers in the electrical wiring in some offices or factories. If there is too much electrical current the circuit breaker will cut off the flow of electrical activity (just like an old-fashioned electrical fuse). To restore the current, you push a button.

Any painful experience involving a shock to the nerves of the bones causes a disturbance in the circuitry in the thalamus. The light touch of Osteomassage on the periosteum causes a temporary overload—trips the circuit breaker—for a split second. Then, the circuit is restored to proper functioning. We essentially erase the history, the memory of the painful experience. It no longer has a negative effect on the body. Releasing a few of these memories seems to be enough to restore the natural movement of the nervous system from sympathetic to parasympathetic.

When the circuit that you have stimulated is cleared out, the blood can flow in the periosteum and you can feel it in your fingertips. If there has been a lot of pain, it takes a longer time to get the pulse. You will also usually notice, as you continue to work on the same bone, the pulses will get stronger and will take less time to come back. Some bones will feel very slow and have a weaker pulse. Other bones on the same person will be faster and stronger. As a person learns how to relax from previous Osteomassage treatments, each time you work on the person, you will generally notice that the pulses are quicker and stronger than at the last treatment. If a person has arthritis, or a lot of stress, or tension in nearby muscles, the pulse can be weak and slow. Therefore, be patient.

Also, for yourself, listening for the pulse will keep you relaxed and heighten your own consciousness. You may find yourself going into light reverie. These dreams, reveries, thoughts, often clear out of your own consciousness an instant before you feel the pulse in the other person. Indeed, as you attune yourself to the other person, you will find that you, yourself, clear out a great deal of your past, even becoming conscious of painful moments that have been hidden away in your own subconscious. That you allow them to come up and that they pass away is enough to clear them so that they no longer create a negative subconscious force. Giving Osteomassage can clear your own mind and bring you closer to your own potential.

When we teach courses, we find that a high percentage of people can come to recognize the pulse after a few practice strokes. There are always a few people who take longer than others. I have seen a few cases where it has taken up to a few hours to be sure of what they should be feeling, as a pulse. You do have to get a feel of it. It will come. After a while you will get an idea of what you are looking for.

Also, as it happens for some people, and it might happen to you, that you sense a pulse but you experience it as coming from your own finger tip, rather than from the periosteum of the other person. That is fine. You can use the pulse in your own finger tip as a guide if you experience it clearly. It is a rather interesting phenomenon. If you feel the pulse in your own finger, it occurs at exactly the same instant as the blood pulses in the periosteum of the person you are working on. This is due to a transmission of energy from the subject's Osteopoint to your finger and this modulates your own pulse. This phenomenon will be observed more clearly with the development of your own experience.

Another thing that can happen as you give Osteomassage is that due to your own relaxation and especially as you move into the awakened state of consciousness that some people experience, you can start to experience time somewhat differently. In different levels of consciousness, time seems to be moving at different rates of speed. Sometimes, you may work for a half an hour and it seems that it has taken only a minute or two though you may think that it must have taken twenty minutes on the clock. So, as you are waiting for the pulse, sometimes it may take a "short" time for it. At other times, it may seem to be taking "forever."

When you can feel the pulse about 85–90 percent of the times you make an Osteomassage stroke, you will be working at a very effective level.

If you have done meditation, tai chi, or yoga for a while, you may start to notice that other things happen in your own body at the instant you feel the pulse in the person that you are working with. This can be valuable for you because you can recognize certain things in yourself at the instant of the pulse which are really indications of a flow of energy in your own parasympathetic nervous system.

If you make more movements on the bones than the suggested single circle, you will not do any harm, but you will not get the clarity you desire in your work on the nervous system.

If you leave your finger on after sensing the pulse, you will notice that there comes another pulse, and another, and another. You will not do any harm, but you will not be helping the other person as effectively as you might.

Always remember, in Osteomassage you are doing more than working on the other person's body. You are also educating their own conscious awareness about tension and relaxation.

When the pulse comes to the periosteum, the person experiences a certain state of mind. Each time you move just after you feel the pulse, you make the other person conscious of what that state of mind feels like. That state of mind cannot be described in words. Every time that you lift your finger an instant after you feel the pulse, you tell the other person that the state of mind that he just experienced is the key to his own relaxation. As he becomes conscious of that state of mind, experienced just at the time of relaxation, he can produce that state of mind more quickly. As he gets used to an open, flowing state of mind in Osteomassage, he will allow himself to enter into deeper and deeper states of relaxation. This relaxed state can give him a different point of view on the problems of his life. Often people get really creative solutions, insights, and intuitive flashes in or just following relaxation.

If you do not wait for the pulse, or if you don't lift your finger just when you feel the pulse, you lose the possibility to educate the other person to recognize the relaxed state of mind. Then he cannot consciously help in the relaxation process. Therefore work with him—give him clear signals of when the pulse comes. Working together with the other person, you will get better results with less time and less effort.

In Osteomassage, using this technique of pulse-feedback, you are not only working on the physical body. You are working on the conscious awareness of the other person. You allow him to expand with confidence, into an experience of his spiritual essence.

Practical Suggestions

Our experience shows that it is best to have the person lie down on a table or on the floor. However, in working on some of the Osteopoints, you can have the person seated on a firm chair.

If the person is lying on his back, it is good to support the back of the head about one and one-half to two and one-half inches. You can use a small pillow. You can also use a book or two wrapped in a towel. You can get a feel for what is a comfortable height—you might use a thick book for one person and a thin book for another. Also, it is good to put something under the back of the knees. By raising the knees from four to six inches you allow a natural relaxation in the lower back. I usually use a regular pillow, folded in half.

To be clothed or not clothed—that is always a question. Other massage forms usually require that the person receiving the massage take his clothing off. In Osteomassage your objective is often to help someone to overcome pain and the situation or the other person's shyness may create an awkward situation if clothing is removed. This could lead to stress or tension.

Fortunately, Osteomassage can be done with the clothing on or the clothing off. You can be effective with the technique through one or more layers of clothing. It is the light stimulation of the nerves of the periosteum that creates the healing effect and a little clothing does not interfere with this. If you have a professional situation to work in, or if the other person is not shy or if personal relationship to the other person makes it natural for you to ask them to take their clothing off and if you feel more comfortable that way, then working directly on the skin is fine. Many people enjoy this. Remember that your point is to help the other person. Be in harmony with his predisposition with regard to being clothed or not clothed. The atmosphere that you create is extremely important.

When you give someone Osteomassage, it is good to have a quiet, peaceful surrounding. Spoken words can be especially distracting to the person you are working on. Of course, if he asks a question, give him an answer. If he wants to tell you what is happening, acknowledge that you have heard what he said. As a rule, I never start a conversation or initiate comments when I am giving the massage. People usually enjoy the Osteomassage and don't say very much.

I usually do my talking with them before they get the massage. Find out how they are feeling, and any problems they have. If it is the first time I have worked on someone I ask why he has come. If he is coming back for another time, I ask him how he has been doing since he last came—and whatever other communication is appropriate. When the massage starts, then I prefer to hold silence unless the person needs to talk about something.

You may find that after you have worked on a person for anywhere from five to twenty minutes, he seems to be asleep. It is not really sleep, but a deep meditative state. He may just enjoy lying there, experiencing the feelings of peace and harmony. It is best to allow him to remain in that state for a few minutes. Some people will get right up as soon as you finish. That is quite all right. Other people will want to stay there for a while.

If you have to interrupt the person while he is in the restful state after the massage, do it gently so that he will have a proper transition back to an active state without losing any of the benefits of the deep relaxation. In a low voice, simply call his name. He will usually blink and turn his head to you. When you see his eyes, tell him that the work for today is over.

In our introductory courses for teaching this technique, the first practice massage usually takes about twenty-five minutes. We usually work on a single bone—the collar bone. People choose to work on the left or the right side.

For people who have never done Osteomassage before, twenty-five minutes on a single bone can sound like a very long time to work on a very small area. But, if you move one-eighth or one-fourth of an inch from one stroke to the next, you may not get from one end of the bone to the other in twenty-five minutes. (If you do finish in less than twenty-five minutes, then start again at one end and work toward the other end.) Concentrating on one bone gives you a chance to learn to recognize the pulse. After you are sure about the feel of the pulse under your finger tip, then you have a basis of experience to work with as you move on to explore other Osteopoints.

It is generally a good idea to balance your work on the right and left sides. If you have worked on a whole bone or on an Osteopoint on one side, then as a rule work on the same area of the skeleton on the other side. This gives you a balance.

When you start your first massage on the collar bone you will find that you can work not only on the surface of the bone under the surface of the skin; you will find also that you can work along the top edge and the bottom edge of the bone. In fact, you will find that in places you can, without forcing, work your fingers onto the back surface of the bone. You can in some places work almost 360° around the collar bone. It produces some very interesting sensations for the other person.

In our beginning courses, we usually take five or ten minutes after the massage for the person receiving the massage and the person giving the massage to talk to each other about what they experienced. People gain insight as to what states of mind and what kinds of experiences accompany this movement from tension to relaxation. This helps them to understand what they are doing. This part of the work is as important in teaching the massage as it is to show the technique and the Osteopoints.

As we discuss things, we remember that everyone is different. Everyone experiences inner states differently. Everyone expresses himself about his inner states in a different way. We learn to appreciate the other person's individuality.

In our courses, working on just one bone for the first massage gives people a clear picture of what a deep, general effect of relaxation can be produced from working on the periosteum, even on such a small area of the body. They can see how effective they can be on the physical, emotional, and mental level of the person they treat with Osteomassage.

The second massage we teach in the beginning courses is called the "Four Corners." Here we take about half an hour to work on a total of four Osteopoints. We use the Osteopoint areas on the collar bone and the corner of the hip bone on the front side of the body, just under the waist (anterior superior iliac spine). Again, we take about half an hour—about seven or eight minutes on each of the four corners. Then as the courses progress, we look at the charts of Osteopoints and start to explore some of the other areas of the body.

Which Points To Choose?

If you are working for the alleviation of pain, especially in arthritis or rheumatism, then work on the bone where the pain is; or, if the pain is in a joint, work on the bones that meet in that joint.

If you want to relax a tense muscle, work on the areas on the bones where that muscle is attached to the bone. If you don't already know about these muscle-bone attachments, you can, with a little effort, study pictures of muscles in an anatomy book to learn where the different muscles attach to the bones; and if you are not a professional health practitioner, one can advise you.

In our advanced courses, we teach special combinations of massage that work in depth on different parts of the body. We have a series of four treatments that free up the rib cage, diaphragm, and other muscles of breathing. We have another series that helps a person work on "grounding"—it concentrates on the hips, knees, ankles, and feet. A third series of massage treatments releases the tensions of the neck, shoulders, and head. We also teach a sequence for the bones of the face.

Many possibilities for creating effective sequences are open to you with the Osteomassage techniques. (Unfortunately, it is beyond the scope of this book to go into these advanced massage sequences in detail.)

Dr. Lawrence has called attention to certain points to work for trouble in the shoulders and for trouble in the lower back.

In the case of shoulder problems, try working on the coracoid process (See photo on page 50).

For lower back, work the sacrum, fifth lumbar vertebra, tailbone, and posterior superior iliac spine. (See page 53).

Osteomassage on Yourself

We have been talking about Osteomassage as a way of working on others, but it is good to know that you can use the same way of working on yourself to bring about deep relaxation, or to help yourself eliminate pains of the bones, joint or muscles.

Now Is the Time To Give It a Try

Bone massage is easy to learn, easy to do, and extremely effective. It produces beneficial results in eliminating or diminishing pain, in bringing deep relaxation and in balancing the nervous system. It works because with a light touch of your finger, you tune into an existing mechanism in the nervous system.

We have gone into some detail in this book to make it possible for you, with professional advice, to give the massage as well as to understand why it works. We have also tried to give you helpful hints to help you handle situations that might arise when you are giving Osteomassage.

It is our hope that you may be able to use this information and this technique to help other people. You can help others to relax from stress and thus gain healthful balance. You can help others to allow the richness of their inner world to unfold to their consciousness. You can help others to be free of debilitating pain so they can do more and more of what they want to do to express themselves with their lives.

If you use yourself as a channel to help other people, you will be helped yourself.

If you wish further clarification or have questions pertaining to the techniques of Osteomassage, you may write to:

Ronald M. Lawrence, M.D.
7535 Laurel Canyon Boulevard
North Hollywood, California 91605